Momfidence

By Priscilla Morales

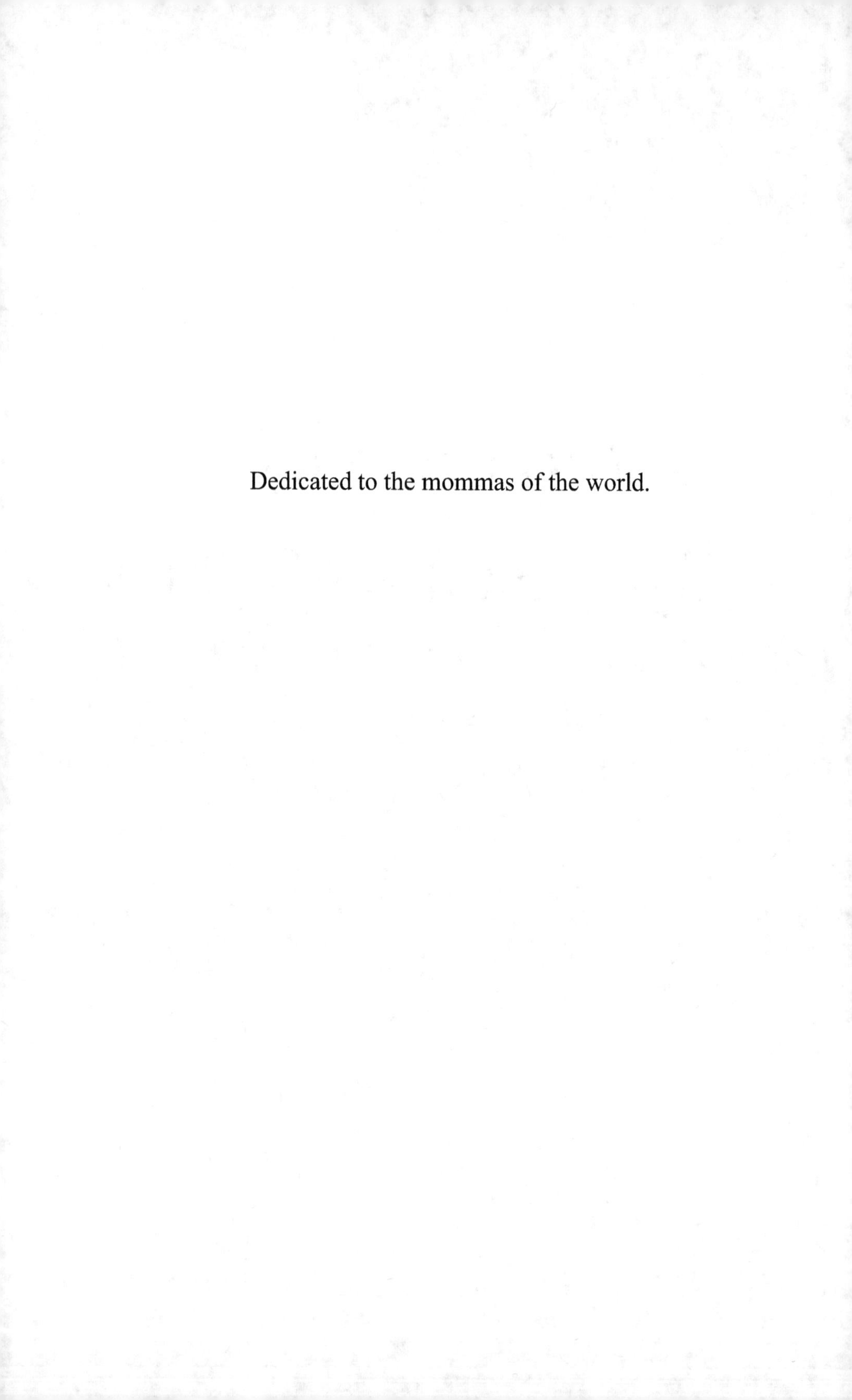

Dedicated to the mommas of the world.

The Phone Call

"Hi. Priscilla, calling to confirm that you are in fact pregnant. Congratulations! Call us back to schedule your next appointment." I found out I was pregnant via voicemail.

I had just celebrated my thirty-fourth birthday. As I put the phone down, my mind was flooded with all kinds of questions: What am I supposed to do now that I am pregnant? Should I stop working out? How soon will I start feeling the pregnancy symptoms? Whom should we tell first? Will I be a good mother? What if my baby does not like me?

I had never really been around newborns or infants. In truth, I had never really envisioned myself as a mother even though my husband and I had planned to be parents. This was a whole new ball game for me. This was no longer the planning stage; this was happening. Once the initial shock from the voicemail wore off a bit, it all started to sink in. My life was never going to be the same again. I was going to be a mother.

I am a planner and a control freak! I love lists and daily planners, so naturally, I dove headfirst into planning for my motherhood journey. I immediately started to download all of the new motherhood apps, and I Googled every question that popped into my head. I signed up for all the mommy classes and began my motherhood research project. I had always been a bit of a bookworm, so I treated these initial stages like I was a student who was about to take a final exam on pregnancy, motherhood, and early childhood development.

I felt like I was drowning in a sea of information. There were thoughts and opinions on everything. I soaked in as much information as I could, but in the end, it didn't give me any real confidence in my ability to be a good mother. Instead, I started to feel anxious about my baby's arrival. I had a tough time sleeping, and the negative thoughts just kept coming. What if something goes wrong? What if my baby does not meet the laid out developmental milestones? What will my body look like after I give birth?

One day, I picked up the phone. I needed to talk to someone who was already a few steps ahead in the motherhood journey. I needed my sister. I laid it all out in what seemed like word vomit. After listening patiently to all my fears and negative self-talk, she gave me the best prenatal advice that I could have received in that moment: "Hey, stop panicking and Google babies in cute costumes!"

It was her way of telling me to relax and focus on all the good things that I was about to experience. That conversation changed my mindset. It was a simple suggestion, but the simple thought of dressing my baby in a super cute outfit made me smile. This positive thought led to more happy thoughts about motherhood. It was the first time that I felt a bit of momfidence.

Change the Channel

Once I made my pregnancy public, it did not take long for other ladies to start sharing their stories. Most of the time, their stories were pleasant and uplifting. However, some of their stories should really be told in high school health classes. They were queasy enough to make anybody practice abstinence for life. I don't think that most people realize the effect that words can have on a pregnant woman, especially one who is experiencing pregnancy for the first time.

One of the best decisions that I made early in my pregnancy was to block out all negative commentary regarding pregnancies and motherhood in general. I decided that their story was theirs and my story would be my own. Their tales of pregnancy terror would have no bearing on what would or would not happen in my life. I developed a type of courage that I had never had before. I became very outspoken when it came to the wellbeing of my child and of myself. Any time that someone would bring up a labor and delivery story that in any way, shape, or form negatively impacted their life, I would simply say, "I thank you for sharing the story with me, but right now, I am just focusing on all the beautiful things that motherhood brings." I felt that adopting this stance at a very early point in my pregnancy helped me transform myself into the person that I knew I needed to become for myself and my baby.

For a long time, I was too shy to ever speak up for myself. I just accepted uncomfortable situations. I avoided confrontation so much that it became an unhealthy habit. The new life growing inside of me gave me the strength, courage, and determination to erase any unnecessary negativity in my own life.

Don't Rub my Belly!

Once my baby bump really popped, it became a hand magnet. Everyone thought that it was okay to touch or rub my belly. Somedays I was okay with belly rubs from my husband and my mom, but I was never okay when strangers reached out to touch my belly without asking. I remember the first time that I had the courage to swat away an unwanted hand. I was having a conversation with a woman who had already made me uncomfortable with her negative baby conversations. In my mind, it happened in slow motion. She reached out and was about to place her hand on my belly when I gently grabbed her hand and pushed it down and said, "No, thank you." I remember the look of surprise on her face and the awkwardness that seemed to follow. I decided that I was okay with the puzzled faces and uncomfortable silence that seemed to fill the room when I said no. Remember, ladies, just because we are now sporting a beautiful baby bump, doesn't mean that we have to accept any type of unwanted commentary or touch.

Muscle Mom

Before becoming pregnant, I led a very active lifestyle. I loved weightlifting and running. After consulting with my health care provider, I decided that I wanted to continue with my workout regimen. I figured I would modify it as my pregnancy progressed and take the necessary steps to stay active and baby safe. However, this did not sit well with others. I was met with critical viewpoints stemming from cultural and personal health beliefs from men and women. Most were genuinely concerned that I might be overexerting myself.

Once again, I was flooded with horror stories of what could potentially happen if I continued to hit the gym.

Concern was coming from all directions, but which advice would I embrace? I decided that I was going to trust my mom instincts.

Seriously, ladies, what it all really boils down to is trusting our instincts when it comes to embracing others' advice. This decision to continue to stay active was an easy one for me. I knew the benefits of staying healthy and exercising. Even though I knew I wanted to remain active, I did not take any decision lightly. I made sure that I took enough time to educate myself on the appropriate nutrition and exercises for a growing baby bump. One of the first gifts that moms give their baby is a healthy body to call home.

The Birth Plan

Okay, so I originally opted for a home water birth. I really wanted to go the all-natural route. This decision was met with a lot of pushback from family and friends. Once again, I met with health providers and decided that this was the best course of action for me, and it was, right up until I went into labor.

Let's just say home water birth was just not the right fit for me. After being in labor for more than a few hours, I opted to head to the hospital for the final show and the epidural shot. People highly criticized both of these choices, but in the end, I made the best choice for myself and my snuggle bug.

As I devoured my postpartum dinner, I decided that I was done explaining my motherhood decisions. After about 30 hours of labor, I successfully pushed out another human. I pushed him out despite any opinions on my health regimen, my homebirth, and my hospital plan. When the time came, my mom instincts kicked in. As I held my newborn son, my momfidence level reached a new high.

This Way and not That Way

Being a mother is the beginning of a beautiful journey, one of strength, bravery, and love. Once my sweet boy was born, I was once again bombarded with motherhood advice. It pretty much started as soon as visitors started to pop in. I opted not to breast feed, mainly because my boobs decided not to produce much milk and my baby was hungry. I did not realize it at the time, but people have very strong opinions about breastfeeding. I also found out that people had strong feelings about mothers co-sleeping and not co-sleeping. Just in case you were wondering, I chose to not co-sleep.

Breast feeding and sleeping arrangements were no doubt hot topics, but the decision of what faith I would choose to raise my son in was by far the most contentious. Allow me to explain. You see, I was raised in a very legalistic religion. About 10 years before I became a mother, I decided that this particular religion was not for me, and I walked away. It had taken many years for my family to accept that I was no longer a part of this faith-based organization, but the idea that I would not be raising my children in this faith troubled them.

Being a new, hormone-filled, sleep-deprived mother is not easy. I was transitioning into a whole new chapter in my life. Adding a bucketful of questions and comments regarding whether or not I would be the reason my child does not receive eternal salvation was not exactly a calming cup of tea.

I had to be unafraid and unwavering in what I knew would be the best decisions for my immediate family's mental and emotional health. I did not have the energy to go into long philosophical debates with family members regarding what they believed was the way to God. I simply said, "I love you, and I appreciate your thoughts, but this is my choice." I would then proceed to change the subject. I didn't want my child to grow up feeling isolated and constantly monitored for what people considered shortcomings in faith. I wanted my baby to feel loved and to know that no matter what happened in life, his mom would never abandon him. My love for my baby made me a stronger and bolder woman.

Mommy's Schedule

I had never envisioned myself as a stay-at-home mother, but that is exactly what I became. I quit my teaching job and embraced the newborn season. We did not have a lot of family around during this time. The family members who did live nearby did their best to check on us, but the truth of the matter was that they had jobs and families of their own. My husband was working long hours, so for the most part, it was just me and my baby.

I do not know exactly how it happened, but it did. My once organized home started to look a bit chaotic. My hair was always in a floppy bun, and my clothes seemed to always have some type of stain on them. I was lonely and overwhelmed with motherhood. Finally, I decided that enough was enough. I kept hearing the voices that predicted my downfall: "Oh, you better enjoy your clean house now. You better enjoy your sleep now. You better enjoy wearing that pretty dress now because once your baby gets here, it is over." I refused to accept their words of doom and gained a little more control over my motherhood chaos.

I decided that I was going to create a master mom schedule. Now, I know it sounds a little crazy at first, but I needed to feel just a little more in control. Now, I know what you are thinking: Priscilla how in the world did you create and stick to a schedule in the middle of newborn season? Well, I had worked as a teacher for a number of years. If there was one thing that I had been trained to do, it was to create organized plans to help make the day run smoothly.

I created a master schedule of everything. I created a color-coded schedule that included feeding time, laundry folding time, reading time, paying bills, and self-care. As crazy as it sounded, it was just my way of taking back control of my life in what seemed an uncontrollable time. I refused to accept that motherhood could not have some semblance of peace. I needed to eat to have energy, and I needed to make sure that when I looked in the mirror, the reflection was someone I recognized and not some crazy looking woman. The master schedule helped me stay organized and returned a bit of my sanity.

Building the Mom Squad

Trust me when I say that you need a mom squad. No one will understand you the way that other mothers will. For example, as much as your husband contributes to the day-to-day activities, he will never understand what it is like to have cracked nipples from breastfeeding. Family members who do not have children will not understand why you are so crazy about staying on nap schedules and why you are so terrified of your kid falling asleep during a 6 pm unnecessary car ride. Having women who understand what you are going through physically, emotionally, and spiritually is an incredible blessing.

Newborn season is now a blur in my mind. I pretty much kept to myself during this time. My husband was working long hours, and for the most part, it was just me and my baby. However, after a while, it started to become a bit lonely. I felt both of us needed to see other faces more regularly. This is when I started to look for mom friends. Thankfully, I did not have to look too far. I had already made a very special friend during my pregnancy. We had bonded over our gym sessions together. Her friendship encouraged me to stay active and healthy throughout my pregnancy. This helped tremendously when it came to maintaining a positive mindset.

Later, around the time that Isaiah was about four months, I set up a blind mom brunch date. I obtained the number of my husband's, coworker's wife who had just had a baby herself. It took me a while, before I worked up the courage to reach out. My text read, "Hey, my name is Priscilla, and I would love to meet you for a baby brunch." I was very happy when she texted me back. Sidenote: making friends with other moms is a little like dating. You smile at other moms at Gymboree or the park, and if the conversation flows, you might ask for her number. You send out the invitation, some will accept it, some will reject it, and sometimes, friends will set you up on blind mom dates. Anyway, back to the story. My blind date mom brunch blossomed into a friendship. Life as a new mom went from being overwhelming to being fun, all because I had friends that I could relate to on a new mom level.

FUN FACT: when you are out with your mom squad, you never have to worry about running out of wipes or diapers. You are never embarrassed if your kid has a meltdown in public. Instead of judgment, you just get, "Yeah, my kid does that, too," and you move on! Life is easier when you surround yourself with mom friends.

Priscilla, where can I meet some fun moms? I've met them at Gymboree, story time, mommy and me classes, mom ministry groups, and of course baby brunch dates. Now, I am not saying that you will hit it off with every mom, but if you are lonely, take a look around. You do not have to walk through motherhood alone. Build your mom squad with moms who uplift and strengthen your momfidence.

Who is Watching the Baby?

Who's watching the baby? This was a question that was asked of me anytime that my child was not glued to my side. I know I am not the only mother who is constantly asked this question. I have been blessed enough to be friends with some powerhouse women. These friends are a combination of working and stay-at-home mothers. All of us are peppered with questions regarding who is watching our children any time that we are not in the same room as them.

Many working mothers tend to feel guilt when returning to work. At least that is how society attempts to make them feel, but why should a mother feel guilty for providing for her children? Why should a woman feel guilty for returning to a career that she worked hard to obtain? A working mom does not love her baby any less just because she returns to work. To constantly question her choices is cruel and unnecessary.

Pizza Night

If a dad is seen picking up a pizza on a weekday, then he is considered a fun dad. If a mom orders takeout, she is more likely to receive judgmental looks. I have received judgmental looks and comments about what I feed my children: "When my children were little, I would always make them a homecooked meal." Regardless of whether this particular individual may or may not be telling the truth, it has zero bearing on my life. Moms are expected to cook, clean, and provide added income for their family. If at any point we fail to do any of these things, hard judgment falls on us. After all, we are at home playing with the baby all day. Why would we not have the time and energy to do it all, right?

It is extremely easy to question our every decision, to wonder if we are making the right choice at every turn. However, it is important to remember that we are doing our best. Our best is enough. If you are a working mom who is working long hours, your children see your effort. If you are a stay-at-home mom who is doing her best to navigate through doctor appointments, playdates, and meals, your children see your effort.

Remember you make certain choices because you know what is best for you and your family. Remembering that I know my family's needs better than anyone else has helped me not shy away from questions that might otherwise make me second-guess my decisions. For example, in the past, I would get upset when people gave unwanted opinions regarding my mothering. Now I simply respond to them by saying something like, "I can see where you are coming from, but this decision is personal and not one that I have made lightly." If they persist in trying to chime in on something that I have deemed none of their business, I just say, "Well, looks like we have different opinions. Let's talk about something else," or I just exit the room if the conversation is getting heated. Momming requires energy, and I no longer have energy to participate in spirited debates over my choices as a mother.

Mom Jeans

I refuse to wear mom jeans. You know, the kind of jeans that go over your belly button and snuggle right under your boobs. I always found them unflattering on me. However, I started to think about why I was obsessing over mom jeans in the first place. Why would they even be a thought in my head? I guess because we are constantly bombarded with images of what the perfect female body should look like. Social media is full of gorgeous looking moms with their perfectly dressed children and their picture-perfect living rooms. Their makeup is perfect, and their hair looks like they just

left the salon. Mom jeans for me represented the opposite of that

picture perfect mom. However, as I continue to walk through my

motherhood journey, I have come to see the beauty that is our ever-

changing bodies.

During my pregnancy, I refused to get on my bathroom scale.

I would only weigh myself during required doctor visits. As long as

my weight stayed healthy, I refused to obsess over it. I knew that it

would be an easy way for me to spiral into a potential unhealthy

behavior. In the past, I used food as a way to feel control over

stressful circumstances. I knew myself enough to know that

weighing myself every day could lead to body issues. I refused to

see my ever-growing baby bump as anything but beautiful.

One of my closest friends, who's also my trainer, was just

amazing during this time because she was also pregnant, so she

understood the days when I just didn't feel like really doing much,

and we would just walk around or do some light weightlifting, It was

fun, and we could relate to each other. During this period, I would

always just tell myself that the future me would thank me for my effort in maintaining a healthy lifestyle during pregnancy, which helped with my confidence. It helped me develop confidence in my physical fitness and my overall well-being. Gifts that I still carry with me every single day. Whether you are wearing mom jeans, a crop top, or a ball gown, remember, your body is beautiful.

Change of Plans

The original plan was to have a home birth. However, things took a bit of a turn for me. I had to make a choice. Should I toss the plan or continue with it? Making quick and tough decisions during childbirth contractions is no easy task. I had to focus, and I had to take charge of what was happening. Some would say that I gave up too easily and that I could have soldiered on and given birth at home. To these individuals, I say if it is not your body, keep your opinions to yourself.

Accepting and Politely Declining Help

In the early stages of motherhood, I felt that asking for help would be admitting that I was failing as a mother. Yes, this type of thinking is ridiculous. I know that now, but at the time, that was just how I felt. I was tired and sleep deprived, my body hurt, and my

hormones were making me go nuts! I am pretty sure I had the baby

blues, but I was too stubborn to admit it. I did not talk about it, and I

didn't ask for help. This was a mistake on my part. There is nothing

wrong with asking for or accepting help from others. Asking for help

can be an act of courage, especially when we are feeling like we are

under a new-mom microscope. I did not want people to see me

looking tired, my laundry loads, or my unwashed baby bottles. I did

not want them to see me crying because I was so exhausted.

Sometimes we have to be momfident enough to say, "Hey guys, I'm

going to need a mom minute." The people who love you and that

matter will be there for you.

Homeschooling Chapter

My daughter was just three months old when the

world shut down. People started to panic. I put on my heavy coat and

ventured out at 4 am just to make sure that I would be one of the first

in line to grab groceries. I remember people rushing inside and

ripping the shopping carts from either side of me. Most of us remember the fights about masks and the arrows that were drawn throughout the food aisles. It was an uncertain and scary time.

I was determined not to allow the chaos that was happening in the world to enter our home. I decided that for the time being, I would homeschool my preschooler. It is still one of the best decisions I have made as a mother.

I looked at various programs, but none of them were quite what I was looking for, so I created my own. I used objects around the house to create fun learning activities for my kids. I used my social media to share our homeschool journey with other moms. This is how "Mommy's Classroom Curriculum" was born. I am forever grateful to have had the opportunity to see my children's development firsthand. I was able to experience the same feeling that a mom gets when her baby walks for the first time or says their first word over and over again. This was truly a blessing for my heart.

Now, with the decision to homeschool came some pushback from well-meaning friends and family. How long will you homeschool? They are eventually going to go back to school, right? Aren't you worried that they will not be properly socialized? I would respond with a simple "We are taking this one academic year at a time. It is working for us now, and that is all that matters."

I also had people randomly quiz my kids about whether they knew their alphabet and primary colors. For the record, my kids were reading by the time they were three and were doing higher grade level math, so yeah, in your face, quizzing people!

After the world settled down a bit, I enrolled Isaiah in the local Carlson Gracie JiuJitsu. I was nervous at first and not sure what to expect. In the beginning, my son was very shy. He would tiptoe around the mat. After a couple of months, I saw his self-confidence skyrocket. This is when I knew that I had made a good decision. As time passed, I noticed that one of the things that gave other kids an advantage on the mats was having a parent who participated in the sport themselves. Now, I had thought about taking self-defense classes many times. Some of my girlfriends had started taking jiu-jitsu classes, and they encouraged me to try it out. I'll be honest: I gave every excuse not to give it a go. It is a contact sport, and I wasn't too keen on getting choked.

It was the desire to give my son the support that he needed that gave me the courage to finally enroll. Being a mom gives you the courage that you need to take on challenges that you would otherwise shy away from. The day I received my first belt stripe, both of my kids were there. Olivia was watching "Daniel Tiger" on my phone, and Isaiah was distracted. At least that is what I thought, but when we arrived back home, Isaiah ran inside and yelled, "Momma got her first stripe! I am so proud of her!"

After a year of training, I hurt my leg. I had not cried like that since childbirth! It was awful, but motherhood also makes you resilient. I took time off to recover, but I had to face the fact that I needed help. Unlike those early days when I struggled alone, I leaned on the people who loved me the most. I have learned that the world will not end if I take time for myself. It was the first time in seven years that I sat down and allowed others to care for me. It was a lesson in self-care. It is not easy, but sometimes we have to force ourselves to sit down and rest. Remember, mommas, if we are to have the strength and energy to take care of our family, we must first take care of ourselves.

Momma Bear Roar

I am that mom! You know the mom that yells from the sidelines. Before becoming a mom, I was a bit of a people-pleasing door mat. Having kids unleashed my momma bear roar. When it comes to my kids, I have zero problems voicing my questions and concerns or, to put it simply, my motherhood enthusiasm. I love my kids. They will never have to wonder whether or not mom will stand up for them. As long as I am around, I will always be their biggest supporter. I have no problem picking up the phone, scheduling an appointment, or knocking on the door of anyone whom I feel needs to hear my momma bear roar.

Protecting my bear cubs is my number one priority. Sometimes, I hear of new moms who feel pressured into allowing their children to participate in activities that they do not feel comfortable with. These activities may be something as simple as allowing their kids to participate in a school field trip, a sleepover, or a playdate. It is important to learn to gage each situation and to remember that every family is different. What works for one family may not necessarily work for another.

For example, our family does not participate in sleepovers. Other families may be okay with sleepovers, but for us, it is not going to happen. Most moms understand and respect our choice, but I have run into moms who get offended when I politely decline. Old me would have felt the need to explain my reasons for my no sleepover policy, but new mom me does not. Remember you do not have to explain your family policies to others unless, of course, you want to. Either way, the final choice is yours because you know what is best for your family.

Back to Work

My husband is an endodontist. After he worked in a corporate office, he was ready to open up his own practice. Now, at first, I wasn't sure that I was even going to be involved in the practice. I loved being a homeschool mom, but circumstances began to shift. Isaiah asked if he could attend school with some of the kids he had befriended in jiujitsu. After seeing his smiling face, I couldn't help but say, "Sure, kid." He walked into class as confident as could be. I, on the other hand, cried all the way home.

I still had my Olivia to preschool homeschool, but the family business needed my support. I took over the marketing aspect of the practice. I would visit various dental practices throughout the city to let them know that our family practice was now open! "Wait … who was watching Olivia?" asked everyone. I took her with me! I packed her snacks and water, I buckled her up, and away we went! We sang songs and took potty breaks. Overall, we made a great team! On the days that I had to do a longer marketing run, I would leave her in our office nursery. My husband and our beloved team would watch her as mom drove around the city. Thank God it all worked out.

Balancing Act

Society puts pressure on moms to do it all. In this chapter of my life, I homeschool, write books, and help run the family business. The truth of the matter is that it was not until Isaiah was enrolled in school and Olivia was potty trained that I was able to focus on other things outside of the home. I didn't do it all at once. The seasons of life change. A lot of times, moms compare their lives to those of other moms who are about nine chapters ahead. Do not compare your toddler season with a mom who has children who are fully potty trained. Do not compare your newborn messy bun and applesauce-covered yoga pants to the mom who is wearing spiked heels and a white dress. Maybe her kids are out of town, she has help, or her kids have graduated from the messy-kid-finger stage. You don't know, so run your own race, Momma.

Now, I am not saying that you cannot get things done, because you can. It just might look a little different from the way you were used to doing things. For example, I have always loved working out. It makes me feel good about myself. However, after I had kids, it takes flexibility and planning for me to get my workout sessions in. When Isaiah was a newborn, he would sleep through my workout, but when he was a toddler, I had to schedule my time during his ever-shortening nap time, and when he stopped napping, I had to move my workout sessions to the early hours of the morning before he popped up. The same thing happened with my writing sessions. I had to carve out time for them. I completed all my writing projects when the family was sleeping.

At first, change can be frustrating because you do not really know what to expect. I am here to remind you that even though it can feel a bit overwhelming at times, things will calm down. Life may look a little different for you for the time being, but you can make things happen. Your body just grew a human. You can do this! Grab your favorite planner and see what can be moved around in your daily routine, and make sure to block out time for the things that make you smile.

Physically Momfident

Now, it is the little things that we do on a daily basis that have a tremendous impact on way that we feel about ourselves. For example, for me to feel somewhat put together, I need a daily workout session. I'm not saying that I get up at the crack of dawn and run ten miles. That has never happened. I do, however, wake up, say my morning prayer, have a 30-minute workout, and take a quick shower. Now again, I am in a new season of life. My kids are sleeping through the night. During my newborn and toddler stages, my routine consisted of catching up on sleep and squeezing in workouts during day naps. However, I never compromised on getting some type of movement in. It was something that I needed.

What do you need to make yourself feel momfident? Is it a workout,

getting your nails done, putting on makeup, or wearing fun jewelry?

Every mom is different. Whatever it is that makes you feel amazing,

carve out the time to do it!

Mother's Mental Health

Now let's talk about our mental health. Only God

knows the countless thoughts and worries that run through our mom

brain. It's nuts! We have to keep track of our kids' daily schedules,

which, depending on their age groups, can include feedings, diaper

changes, playdates, school pickups, school drop offs, after-school

sports, doctor's appointments, birthdays, parent-teacher conferences,

and special holiday activities, and of course, we have to keep track

of our housekeeping schedule, tutoring, car maintenance, traffic, and

commutes. This does not include a working mom's thoughts. That's

a whole other load that includes more deadlines.

No wonder moms hide out in the bathroom just to get a few

minutes of peace, so how do we keep a healthy mind space in this

crazy jumble of thoughts? This is what works for me. Before I even get out of bed, I say a morning prayer. This helps me focus my mind before my feet even touch the floor. Then I get my body moving. I give myself enough time in the morning for a quick workout. During this time, I usually listen to one of my favorite podcasts, usually the episodes that remind me to keep a positive mindset throughout the day.

I do not check my email, social media, or the news until I am showered, changed, and ready to start my day. This decision was a turning point for me. It helped me start and keep a positive mindset. Some things that my friends love doing to keep their mind peaceful include journaling, mediation, rock painting, knitting, and mom ministry groups. Do whatever activity you feel will contribute to your mental health. The way you feel about yourself will have a direct impact on the way that you interact with others, especially the tiny humans who require our attention.

Romance

Wait, Priscilla, what about your romantic relationship with your husband? How do you keep it spicy when you are flooded with mom duties? Well, ladies, like most things in this season, date night must be scheduled and made a priority. Now, not everyone has childcare readily available. Sometimes date nights will have to take place at home after the kids have gone to bed. Enjoy a meal together, snuggle up under a blanket and watch a movie, or make it a point to hold hands when you are going on a family stroll. The important thing is that you spend quality time together.

Also, it is crucial that you dress for date night, even a stay-at-home date night. Remember when you were dating. No way would you go on a date in dirty sweatpants and with greasy hair and an unwashed face. I'm not saying that you have to wear spiked heels, but if you do not feel sexy, chances are you are not giving date night vibes. The same is true for your partner. You would never go on a second date with someone who showed up looking like they just pulled clothes out of a hamper or stared at their phone during dinner, so whether you have been married for two years or a decade, make sure that you prioritize your relationship with your significant other.

Conclusion

Take a moment, look in the mirror, and say, "I am a good mom." Motherhood is not easy, but you are doing great. Yes, there are days when you might have to order pizza for dinner or turn on the television for a few added minutes of quiet time. You are doing your best, and your best is enough.

Dear Diary,

I am a good mom.

Yesterday I_______________

Today I ________________

Tomorrow I will ___________

Yes, I am a good mom.

List 5 things that you love about yourself:

1.

2.

3.

4.

5

Hey, mom squad, thank you for sharing the motherhood journey with me.

Love Always,

Priscilla

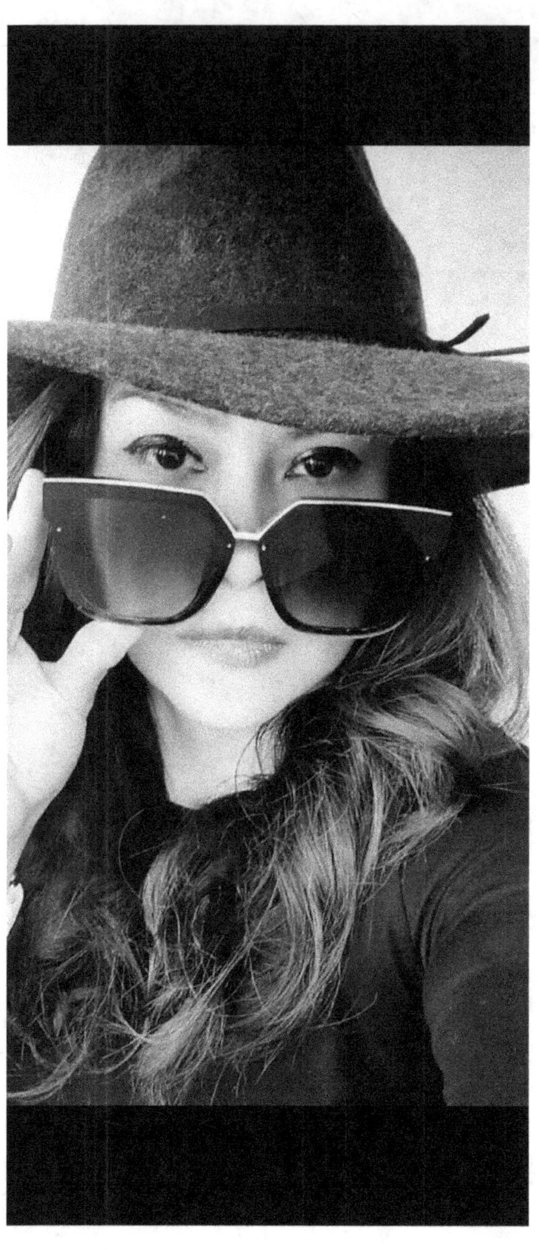

MOMFIDENCE!

www.ingramcontent.com/pod-product-compliance
Lightning Source LLC
Chambersburg PA
CBHW070751260726
48660CB00007B/3064